TRYING TO CONCEIVE? HERE'S WHAT YOU NEED TO KNOW

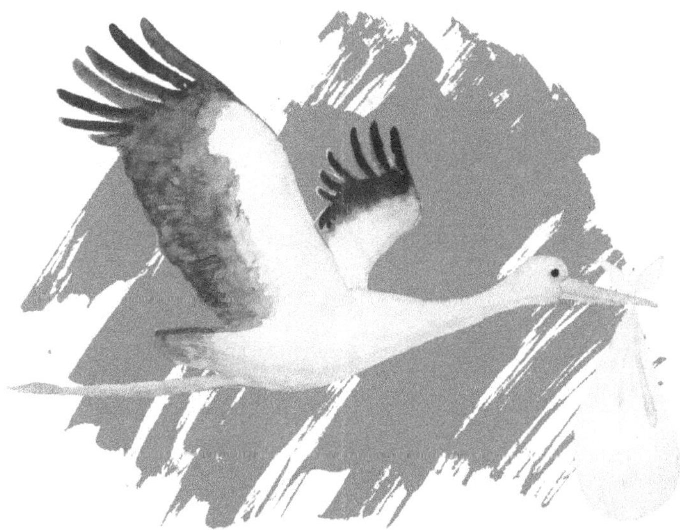

Aurora Brooks

xspurts.com

Created by <u>BabyDreamers.net</u>

Free Book Offer:
Get How to be a Super Mom For Free

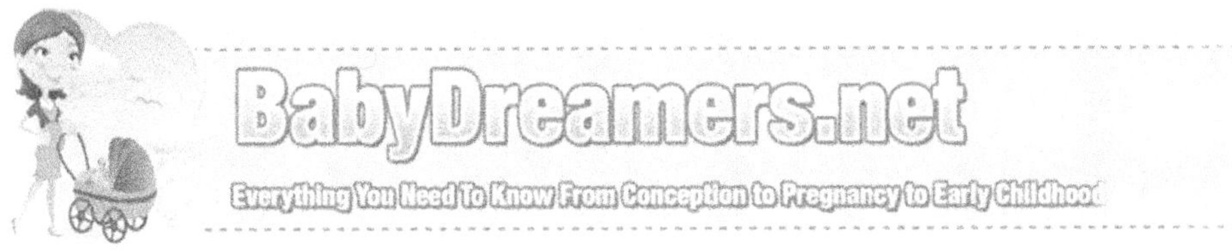

A Short Read is a type of book that is designed to be read in one quick sitting.

These no fluff books are perfect for people who want an overview about a subject in a short period of time.

Table of Contents

MANAGING ANXIETY

SEEKING SUPPORT

FREQUENTLY ASKED QUESTIONS

Have Questions / Comments?

Get How To Be A Super Mom 100% FREE

Trying to Conceive? Here's What You Need to Know

Trying to conceive can be an exciting and sometimes challenging journey. If you're hoping to start a family, it's important to have a comprehensive understanding of the factors that can impact your fertility. This guide is designed to provide you with the knowledge and information you need to navigate the process of trying to conceive.

Fertility awareness is a crucial aspect of your journey. Understanding your menstrual cycle and tracking your ovulation can greatly increase your chances of getting pregnant. By knowing when you're most fertile, you can time intercourse accordingly. We'll delve into the different phases of your menstrual cycle and provide you with tips on how to track your ovulation effectively.

In addition to fertility awareness, there are various lifestyle factors that can impact your fertility. Your diet, exercise routine, stress levels, and exposure to harmful substances can all play a role in your ability to conceive. We'll explore the importance of healthy eating for fertility, the role of exercise in enhancing fertility, effective stress management techniques, and the substances you should avoid when trying to conceive.

Furthermore, we'll discuss common medical conditions that can affect fertility. Conditions such as polycystic ovary syndrome (PCOS) and endometriosis can present challenges when trying to conceive. Understanding these conditions and the available treatment options can help you make informed decisions about your fertility journey.

If you're struggling to conceive, it may be time to seek medical help. We'll guide you through the process of consulting a fertility specialist, from the initial evaluation to diagnostic tests. We'll also explore the causes of female and male infertility, as well as the various treatment options available, including fertility medications, intrauterine insemination (IUI), and in vitro fertilization (IVF).

Lastly, we'll touch on alternative approaches to fertility, such as acupuncture, herbal supplements, and mind-body therapies. These complementary therapies can offer additional support and potentially enhance your fertility journey. We'll also address the emotional challenges that can arise when trying to conceive, including coping with disappointment, managing anxiety, and seeking support.

By arming yourself with knowledge and understanding, you can navigate the journey of trying to conceive with confidence. Whether you're just starting out or have been trying for some time, this comprehensive guide will provide you with the information you need to make informed decisions and optimize your chances of achieving a successful pregnancy.

Understanding Your Menstrual Cycle

Understanding Your Menstrual Cycle

When it comes to trying to conceive, understanding your menstrual cycle is crucial. Your menstrual cycle is the monthly hormonal cycle that prepares your body for pregnancy. It consists of several phases, each with its own unique characteristics and functions. By tracking your menstrual cycle, you can identify the most fertile days and increase your chances of getting pregnant.

The menstrual cycle is divided into four main phases: the menstrual phase, the follicular phase, ovulation, and the luteal phase. Let's take a closer look at each phase:

- **Menstrual Phase:** This is the phase when you experience your period. It typically lasts for 3-7 days and marks the shedding of the uterine lining.
- **Follicular Phase:** Following your period, the follicular phase begins. During this phase, follicles in your ovaries start to mature and produce estrogen, preparing the body for ovulation.
- **Ovulation:** Ovulation is the release of a mature egg from the ovary. This usually occurs around the middle of your cycle. It is the most fertile time, as the egg can be fertilized by sperm for about 24-48 hours after its release.
- **Luteal Phase:** After ovulation, the luteal phase begins. During this phase, the ruptured follicle transforms into a structure called the corpus luteum, which produces progesterone. Progesterone helps prepare the uterus for possible implantation of a fertilized egg.

To maximize your chances of getting pregnant, it's important to track your ovulation. There are several methods you can use to determine when you are ovulating, such as tracking your basal body temperature, monitoring changes in cervical mucus, or using ovulation predictor kits. By identifying your fertile window, you can time intercourse to coincide with ovulation and increase your chances of conception.

Understanding your menstrual cycle and tracking ovulation can greatly increase your chances of getting pregnant. By knowing when you are most fertile, you can optimize your attempts to conceive and take proactive steps towards starting or expanding your family.

Optimizing Your Fertility

When it comes to trying to conceive, there are several lifestyle factors that can significantly impact your fertility. By making certain changes and adopting healthy habits, you can increase your chances of getting pregnant. Let's take a closer look at some of these factors:

- **Diet:** A balanced and nutritious diet plays a crucial role in optimizing fertility. Make sure to include a variety of fruits, vegetables, whole grains, lean proteins, and healthy fats in your meals. Certain nutrients, such as folate, iron, and omega-3 fatty acids, are particularly beneficial for fertility.
- **Exercise:** Regular physical activity is not only essential for overall health but also for fertility. Engaging in moderate exercise for at least 30 minutes a day can help regulate hormones, improve blood circulation to the reproductive organs, and enhance fertility. Aim for a combination of cardio exercises, strength training, and yoga.
- **Stress Management:** High levels of stress can have a negative impact on fertility. Find effective stress management techniques that work for you, such as meditation, deep breathing exercises, or engaging in activities that you enjoy. Taking time to relax and unwind can help balance hormones and increase your chances of conceiving.
- **Avoiding Harmful Substances:** Certain substances can impair fertility and harm your chances of getting pregnant. It's important to avoid tobacco, alcohol, and excessive caffeine, as they can negatively affect both male and female fertility. Additionally, some medications may also interfere with conception, so consult with your healthcare provider about any medications you are taking.

By focusing on these lifestyle factors and making positive changes, you can optimize your fertility and increase your chances of conceiving. Remember that every individual is unique, and it may take time to see results. Be patient, stay committed to a healthy lifestyle, and consult with a healthcare professional for personalized advice.

Healthy Eating for Fertility

Healthy Eating for Fertility

When it comes to trying to conceive, maintaining a healthy diet is crucial. A balanced diet not only supports overall health but also plays a significant role in fertility. By fueling your body with the right nutrients, you can optimize your reproductive system and increase your chances of getting pregnant.

One nutrient that is particularly important for fertility is folate. This B-vitamin is essential for the development of the baby's neural tube and can help prevent birth defects. Good sources of folate include leafy green vegetables, citrus fruits, and fortified cereals.

In addition to folate, iron is another nutrient that plays a key role in fertility. Iron helps carry oxygen to the reproductive organs and is necessary for the production of healthy eggs. Foods rich in iron include lean meats, beans, spinach, and fortified grains.

Omega-3 fatty acids are also beneficial for fertility. These healthy fats have been shown to improve hormone production, regulate the menstrual cycle, and support overall reproductive health. Good sources of omega-3 fatty acids include fatty fish like salmon and sardines, flaxseeds, and walnuts.

When planning your meals, aim for a variety of nutrient-dense foods. Incorporate plenty of fruits, vegetables, whole grains, lean proteins, and healthy fats into your diet. It's also important to stay hydrated by drinking plenty of water throughout the day.

In addition to eating a healthy diet, consider taking a prenatal vitamin to ensure you're getting all the necessary nutrients for fertility. Your healthcare provider can recommend a prenatal vitamin that meets your specific needs.

Remember, healthy eating is just one piece of the fertility puzzle. It's important to combine a nutritious diet with other lifestyle factors, such as regular exercise, stress management, and avoiding harmful substances, to optimize your chances of conceiving.

The Role of Exercise

Exercise plays a crucial role in enhancing fertility and increasing the chances of conception for women. Regular physical activity not only promotes overall health and well-being but also positively impacts reproductive function. Engaging in the right types of exercises can optimize fertility and improve the chances of getting pregnant.

When it comes to exercise and fertility, it's important to strike a balance. While moderate exercise can be beneficial, excessive or intense workouts may have a negative impact on reproductive health. It's essential to find the right balance and avoid overexertion.

So, which types of exercises are recommended for women trying to conceive? Low-impact exercises such as walking, swimming, and cycling are excellent choices. These activities provide cardiovascular benefits without putting excessive stress on the body.

Yoga and Pilates are also great options as they help improve flexibility, reduce stress, and promote relaxation.

It's important to note that every woman is different, and what works for one person may not work for another. It's recommended to consult with a healthcare professional or a fertility specialist to determine the most suitable exercise routine based on individual needs and health conditions.

In addition to exercise, maintaining a healthy lifestyle is essential for optimizing fertility. This includes following a balanced diet, managing stress levels, and avoiding harmful substances. By incorporating exercise into your daily routine and adopting a healthy lifestyle, you can enhance your fertility and increase your chances of conceiving.

Managing Stress for Conception

Managing Stress for Conception

When it comes to trying to conceive, managing stress is crucial. High levels of stress can negatively impact fertility by disrupting hormonal balance and affecting ovulation. Fortunately, there are effective stress management techniques that can help reduce the negative impact of stress on fertility.

One of the most important things you can do is to prioritize self-care. This includes taking time for yourself, engaging in activities that bring you joy and relaxation, and practicing self-compassion. It's essential to listen to your body and give yourself permission to rest and recharge.

In addition to self-care, there are various stress reduction techniques that you can incorporate into your daily routine. Deep breathing exercises, meditation, and mindfulness practices can help calm the mind and relax the body. These techniques can be especially helpful during stressful moments or when you find yourself feeling overwhelmed.

Another effective way to manage stress is through physical activity. Engaging in regular exercise not only helps release endorphins, which are natural mood boosters, but it also promotes better sleep and overall well-being. Find an exercise routine that you enjoy, whether it's going for a walk, practicing yoga, or engaging in a sport.

It's also important to establish healthy boundaries and learn to say no when necessary. Prioritize your emotional well-being and avoid taking on too many responsibilities or commitments that may increase stress levels. Remember, it's okay to ask for help and delegate tasks when needed.

Lastly, consider seeking support from loved ones or joining a support group for individuals experiencing similar challenges. Talking about your feelings and concerns with others who understand can provide a sense of validation and comfort. If you find that stress is significantly impacting your daily life and ability to cope, consider seeking professional help from a therapist or counselor who specializes in fertility-related issues.

By implementing these stress management techniques, you can create a more balanced and supportive environment for conception. Remember, taking care of your emotional well-being is just as important as taking care of your physical health when trying to conceive.

Avoiding Harmful Substances

When trying to conceive, it's important to be mindful of the substances you expose your body to. Certain substances can have a negative impact on fertility and increase the risk of pregnancy complications. Here are some substances that you should avoid:

- Tobacco: Smoking tobacco has been linked to decreased fertility in both men and women. It can also increase the risk of miscarriage and ectopic pregnancy.
- Alcohol: Consuming alcohol can impair fertility and increase the risk of birth defects. It's best to avoid alcohol altogether when trying to conceive.
- Caffeine: While moderate caffeine consumption is generally safe, excessive intake can interfere with conception. It's recommended to limit caffeine intake to 200 milligrams per day, which is roughly equivalent to one cup of coffee.
- Certain Medications: Some medications can interfere with fertility or harm a developing fetus. It's important to consult with your healthcare provider about any medications you are taking or plan to take while trying to conceive.

By avoiding these substances, you can create a healthier environment for conception and increase your chances of a successful pregnancy. It's also important to remember that both partners should make an effort to avoid these substances, as they can affect male fertility as well.

Understanding Reproductive Health

Understanding Reproductive Health

Reproductive health plays a crucial role in a woman's ability to conceive. There are several common reproductive health issues that can impact fertility, including polycystic ovary syndrome (PCOS) and endometriosis. It's important to have a thorough understanding of these conditions and their effects on fertility in order to seek appropriate treatment and support.

Polycystic ovary syndrome (PCOS) is a hormonal disorder that affects many women of reproductive age. It is characterized by the presence of multiple cysts on the ovaries, irregular menstrual cycles, and high levels of androgen hormones. PCOS can disrupt ovulation and make it more difficult to conceive. Women with PCOS may also experience symptoms such as weight gain, acne, and excessive hair growth. Treatment options for PCOS may include lifestyle changes, medication to regulate hormones, and assisted reproductive technologies.

Endometriosis is another common reproductive health issue that can affect fertility. It occurs when the tissue that normally lines the uterus grows outside of it, often on the ovaries, fallopian tubes, or other pelvic organs. This condition can cause inflammation, scar tissue, and the formation of adhesions, which can interfere with the normal functioning of the reproductive organs. Symptoms of endometriosis may include pelvic pain, painful periods, and infertility. Treatment options for endometriosis include medication, surgery, and assisted reproductive technologies.

By understanding these common reproductive health issues, individuals can be better equipped to navigate their fertility journey and seek appropriate medical intervention when necessary. It's important to consult with a healthcare professional to receive an accurate diagnosis and personalized treatment plan. Remember, knowledge is power when it comes to reproductive health and fertility.

Polycystic Ovary Syndrome (PCOS)

Polycystic Ovary Syndrome (PCOS) is a hormonal disorder that affects women of reproductive age. It is characterized by the presence of multiple cysts on the ovaries, irregular menstrual cycles, and high levels of androgens (male hormones) in the body. PCOS is a common condition that can significantly impact fertility.

One of the main symptoms of PCOS is irregular or absent menstrual periods. Women with PCOS may experience infrequent or prolonged menstrual cycles, making it difficult to predict ovulation and conceive. Other symptoms include excessive hair growth (hirsutism), acne, weight gain, and difficulty losing weight.

The exact cause of PCOS is not fully understood, but it is believed to involve a combination of genetic and environmental factors. Insulin resistance, a condition in which the body's cells do not respond properly to insulin, is often associated with PCOS. This can lead to elevated insulin levels, which in turn stimulate the ovaries to produce more androgens.

Treatment options for PCOS aim to manage the symptoms and improve fertility. Lifestyle changes, such as maintaining a healthy weight through diet and exercise, can help regulate menstrual cycles and improve insulin sensitivity. Medications, such as oral contraceptives, anti-androgens, and insulin-sensitizing drugs, may also be prescribed to manage symptoms and restore hormonal balance.

In some cases, fertility treatments may be necessary for women with PCOS who are trying to conceive. These treatments may include ovulation induction with medications, such as clomiphene citrate or letrozole, to stimulate egg production. In more severe cases, in vitro fertilization (IVF) may be recommended to bypass any ovulation or fertility issues.

It is important for women with PCOS to work closely with a healthcare provider who specializes in reproductive health. They can provide personalized guidance and treatment options to help manage the symptoms of PCOS and increase the chances of successful conception.

Endometriosis

Endometriosis is a common condition that can have a significant impact on fertility. It occurs when the tissue that normally lines the uterus, called the endometrium, grows outside of the uterus. This abnormal growth can cause inflammation, scarring, and the formation of adhesions, which can interfere with the normal functioning of the reproductive organs.

One of the main challenges of endometriosis is that it can cause infertility. The presence of endometrial tissue outside of the uterus can affect the quality of the eggs, the function of the fallopian tubes, and the implantation of the fertilized egg in the uterus. This can make it more difficult for women with endometriosis to conceive naturally.

Fortunately, there are treatment options available to manage endometriosis and improve fertility. The specific treatment approach will depend on the severity of the symptoms and the individual's reproductive goals. Hormonal therapies, such as birth control pills or gonadotropin-releasing hormone (GnRH) agonists, may be prescribed to suppress the growth of endometrial tissue and alleviate symptoms. In some cases, surgery may be recommended to remove endometrial implants, adhesions, or cysts.

It's important for individuals with endometriosis who are trying to conceive to work closely with a fertility specialist. They can provide guidance on the most appropriate treatment options and help optimize the chances of achieving a successful pregnancy. Additionally, support groups and counseling services can offer emotional support and coping strategies for individuals dealing with the emotional and physical challenges of endometriosis and infertility.

When to Seek Medical Help

When it comes to trying to conceive, there may come a point where seeking medical help becomes necessary. If you have been actively trying to get pregnant for a year without success, or if you are over the age of 35 and have been trying for six months, it's time to consult a fertility specialist. These professionals are trained in diagnosing and treating fertility issues, and they can provide valuable guidance and support throughout your journey.

During your initial evaluation with a fertility specialist, you can expect a thorough assessment of your reproductive health. This may involve a series of diagnostic tests to identify any underlying issues that could be affecting your fertility. These tests may include blood work to check hormone levels, imaging tests to evaluate the reproductive organs, and a semen analysis for your partner.

Based on the results of these tests, your fertility specialist will be able to provide you with a diagnosis and recommend appropriate treatment options. It's important to remember that fertility treatments are not one-size-fits-all, and what works for one person may not work for another. Your fertility specialist will work closely with you to develop a personalized treatment plan tailored to your specific needs and goals.

Understanding Female Infertility

Female infertility can be caused by various factors, including ovulation disorders, fallopian tube blockages, and uterine abnormalities. Let's take a closer look at each of these causes:

- **Ovulation Disorders:** One of the most common causes of female infertility is ovulation disorders. These disorders can prevent the release of mature eggs from the ovaries, making it difficult for fertilization to occur. Hormonal imbalances, polycystic ovary syndrome (PCOS), and thyroid problems are some of the conditions that can disrupt ovulation.
- **Fallopian Tube Blockages:** The fallopian tubes play a crucial role in transporting eggs from the ovaries to the uterus. Blockages or damage to the fallopian tubes can prevent the sperm from reaching the egg or the fertilized

egg from reaching the uterus. Pelvic inflammatory disease, endometriosis, and previous surgeries can lead to fallopian tube blockages.

- **Uterine Abnormalities:** The uterus provides a nurturing environment for the fertilized egg to implant and develop into a fetus. Structural abnormalities in the uterus, such as fibroids, polyps, or adhesions, can interfere with implantation or cause recurrent miscarriages.

It's important to consult with a fertility specialist if you suspect you may be experiencing female infertility. They can conduct diagnostic tests to identify the specific cause and recommend appropriate treatment options.

Understanding Male Infertility

Understanding Male Infertility

Male infertility can be caused by a variety of factors, including sperm abnormalities, hormonal imbalances, and genetic conditions. These factors can significantly impact a man's ability to father a child. Understanding the potential causes of male infertility is crucial in seeking appropriate medical help and exploring treatment options.

Sperm Abnormalities

Sperm abnormalities are a common cause of male infertility. These abnormalities can include low sperm count, poor sperm motility (movement), and abnormal sperm shape. These issues can make it difficult for sperm to reach and fertilize an egg, resulting in infertility. Various factors can contribute to sperm abnormalities, such as genetic factors, hormonal imbalances, and lifestyle choices like smoking or excessive alcohol consumption.

Hormonal Imbalances

Hormonal imbalances can also play a role in male infertility. Hormones like testosterone and follicle-stimulating hormone (FSH) are essential for sperm production. If there is an imbalance in these hormones, it can affect the quality and quantity of sperm. Conditions like hypogonadism, where the testes do not produce enough testosterone, can contribute to male infertility. Hormonal imbalances can be caused by genetic conditions, certain medications, or underlying health issues.

Genetic Conditions

Genetic conditions can also be a factor in male infertility. Certain genetic disorders can affect the development and function of the reproductive system, leading to infertility. Examples of genetic conditions that can contribute to male infertility include Klinefelter syndrome, Y chromosome deletions, and cystic fibrosis gene mutations. It is important for individuals with a family history of genetic conditions to seek genetic counseling and testing to understand their risk of infertility.

In conclusion, male infertility can be caused by various factors, including sperm abnormalities, hormonal imbalances, and genetic conditions. Understanding these factors is essential in diagnosing and treating male infertility. If you are struggling with infertility, it is important to consult a fertility specialist who can provide personalized guidance and treatment options based on your specific situation.

Fertility Treatments

Fertility Treatments

When natural conception proves challenging, there are a variety of fertility treatment options available to assist couples in their journey towards parenthood. These treatments are designed to address specific fertility issues and increase the chances of achieving a successful pregnancy. Here, we will explore some of the most common fertility treatment options, including medications, intrauterine insemination (IUI), and in vitro fertilization (IVF).

Medications:

Medications are often the first line of treatment for couples struggling with fertility issues. These medications work by stimulating ovulation in women or improving sperm production and quality in men. Common medications used for fertility treatment include:

- Clomiphene citrate
- Letrozole
- Gonadotropins
- Metformin

It's important to note that these medications should only be taken under the guidance of a fertility specialist, as they can have side effects and require careful monitoring.

Intrauterine Insemination (IUI):

IUI, also known as artificial insemination, is a fertility treatment that involves placing sperm directly into the uterus to increase the chances of fertilization. This procedure is often recommended for couples with mild fertility issues or unexplained infertility. The process typically involves the following steps:

1. Ovulation induction: The woman may be prescribed fertility medications to stimulate the ovaries and promote the development of multiple eggs.
2. Sperm preparation: The male partner provides a semen sample, which is then washed and concentrated to separate the healthy sperm from the seminal fluid.
3. Insemination: The concentrated sperm is carefully inserted into the woman's uterus using a thin catheter.
4. Monitoring and support: The woman may be advised to rest for a short period after the procedure, and the fertility specialist will monitor her progress through blood tests and ultrasounds.

In Vitro Fertilization (IVF):

IVF is a more advanced fertility treatment that involves fertilizing the eggs with sperm in a laboratory setting before transferring the resulting embryos into the woman's uterus. This procedure is often recommended for couples with more complex fertility issues, such as blocked fallopian tubes, severe male factor infertility, or previous unsuccessful fertility treatments. The IVF process typically includes the following stages:

1. Ovarian stimulation: The woman undergoes hormone injections to stimulate the ovaries and produce multiple mature eggs.
2. Egg retrieval: The eggs are retrieved from the woman's ovaries using a minimally invasive procedure called transvaginal ultrasound-guided aspiration.
3. Fertilization: The retrieved eggs are combined with sperm in a laboratory dish to facilitate fertilization.
4. Embryo development: The fertilized eggs, now embryos, are cultured in a laboratory for a few days to allow for optimal development.
5. Embryo transfer: One or more embryos are transferred into the woman's uterus using a thin catheter.
6. Monitoring and support: The woman will be closely monitored for signs of pregnancy, and if successful, she will continue to receive support throughout the early stages of pregnancy.

It's important to remember that fertility treatments should be discussed with a fertility specialist who can provide personalized recommendations based on individual circumstances. These treatments can be emotionally and physically demanding, but they offer hope and the possibility of fulfilling the dream of starting a family.

Fertility Medications

When it comes to trying to conceive, fertility medications can play a crucial role in stimulating ovulation and improving fertility. These medications are commonly prescribed by fertility specialists and can help increase the chances of pregnancy for individuals facing ovulation disorders or other fertility issues.

There are several types of fertility medications available, each with its own mechanism of action and potential side effects. Let's take a closer look at some of the common medications used in fertility treatments:

- **Clomiphene Citrate:** This oral medication is often the first line of treatment for women with ovulation disorders. It works by stimulating the release of hormones that trigger ovulation. However, it may cause side effects such as hot flashes, mood swings, and bloating.
- **Letrozole:** Another oral medication, letrozole, is sometimes used as an alternative to clomiphene citrate. It works by inhibiting estrogen production, which can stimulate ovulation. Side effects may include headaches, dizziness, and nausea.
- **Gonadotropins:** These injectable medications contain follicle-stimulating hormone (FSH) and luteinizing hormone (LH), which directly stimulate the ovaries to produce eggs. Gonadotropins are often used in combination with other fertility treatments and may have side effects such as abdominal discomfort and bloating.

It's important to note that fertility medications should only be taken under the guidance of a fertility specialist. They will carefully monitor your response to the medications and adjust the dosage as needed to minimize side effects and maximize the chances of success.

Success rates with fertility medications vary depending on various factors, including the underlying cause of infertility and the individual's overall health. It's essential to have realistic expectations and understand that fertility medications may not work for everyone. However, they can significantly improve the chances of ovulation and pregnancy for many individuals.

If you're considering fertility medications, it's crucial to discuss the potential risks, benefits, and side effects with your fertility specialist. They will be able to provide personalized recommendations based on your specific situation and help you make informed decisions about your fertility journey.

Intrauterine Insemination (IUI)

IUI, also known as intrauterine insemination, is a fertility treatment that can increase the chances of pregnancy by placing sperm directly into the uterus. This procedure is often recommended for couples who are experiencing difficulties conceiving due to various reasons.

During an IUI procedure, the male partner's sperm is collected and processed in a laboratory to separate the healthy sperm from the semen. The processed sperm is then inserted into the uterus using a thin catheter, which is inserted through the cervix. This allows the sperm to bypass any potential barriers and increases the chances of fertilization.

IUI is often recommended for couples who have been trying to conceive for a certain period of time without success. It can be a suitable option for couples with unexplained infertility, mild male factor infertility, or cervical issues that may hinder sperm from reaching the uterus. Additionally, IUI may be recommended for couples using donor sperm or for those undergoing fertility treatments such as ovulation induction.

Before undergoing an IUI procedure, both partners may need to undergo certain tests to ensure that they are suitable candidates. These tests may include semen analysis, blood tests to check hormone levels, and an evaluation of the female partner's uterus and fallopian tubes.

It's important to note that IUI is not suitable for everyone, and the success rates can vary depending on various factors such as age, overall health, and the underlying cause of infertility. Your fertility specialist will be able to provide you with personalized guidance and recommendations based on your specific situation.

Overall, IUI can be a less invasive and more affordable fertility treatment compared to other options such as in vitro fertilization (IVF). It is a procedure that offers hope to couples who are struggling to conceive and can significantly increase the chances of achieving a successful pregnancy.

In Vitro Fertilization (IVF)

Are you considering in vitro fertilization (IVF) as a fertility treatment option? In this section, we will provide you with insights into the IVF process, from ovarian stimulation to embryo transfer, as well as important information about success rates and potential risks.

The IVF process typically begins with ovarian stimulation, where medications are used to stimulate the ovaries to produce multiple mature eggs. This is done to increase the chances of successful fertilization. During this phase, you will be closely monitored through blood tests and ultrasounds to track the development of your eggs.

Once the eggs have reached maturity, they will be retrieved through a minor surgical procedure called egg retrieval. This procedure is usually performed under sedation or anesthesia to ensure your comfort. The retrieved eggs are then fertilized with sperm in a laboratory, either through traditional IVF or intracytoplasmic sperm injection (ICSI), depending on the specific circumstances.

After fertilization, the resulting embryos are cultured in a laboratory for a few days, typically between three to five days. During this time, the embryos are carefully monitored for their development and quality. The best quality embryos are selected for transfer into the uterus.

Embryo transfer is a relatively simple procedure where the selected embryos are placed into the uterus using a thin catheter. This is usually done without anesthesia and is generally painless. After the transfer, you will be advised to rest for a short period before resuming your normal activities.

It's important to note that the success rates of IVF can vary depending on various factors, such as age, underlying fertility issues, and the quality of embryos. Your fertility specialist will discuss your individual chances of success based on your specific circumstances.

While IVF can be an effective fertility treatment, it's essential to be aware of potential risks and complications. These may include multiple pregnancies, ovarian hyperstimulation syndrome (OHSS), and the emotional and financial stress associated with the treatment. Your fertility specialist will provide you with detailed information about the potential risks and help you make an informed decision.

If you are considering IVF, it's crucial to consult with a fertility specialist who can guide you through the entire process, answer your questions, and provide the necessary support. Remember, every fertility journey is unique, and understanding the IVF process and its potential outcomes will empower you to make informed decisions about your fertility treatment.

Alternative Approaches to Fertility

Alternative approaches to fertility offer individuals and couples additional options to enhance their chances of conceiving. These approaches, including acupuncture, herbal supplements, and mind-body therapies, have gained popularity for their potential benefits in supporting fertility.

Acupuncture is a traditional Chinese medicine practice that involves the insertion of thin needles into specific points on the body. It is believed to improve fertility by promoting blood flow to the reproductive organs, balancing hormones, and reducing stress. Many individuals have reported positive outcomes and increased fertility rates after incorporating acupuncture into their fertility journey.

Herbal supplements are another alternative approach that individuals may consider when trying to conceive. Certain herbs, such as chasteberry, maca root, and red raspberry leaf, are believed to support reproductive health and hormone balance. However, it is important to consult with a healthcare professional before starting any herbal supplements, as they may interact with medications or have potential side effects.

Mind-body therapies, such as yoga, meditation, and visualization, can also be beneficial for individuals navigating the fertility journey. These practices help reduce stress, promote relaxation, and create a positive mindset. By incorporating these techniques into their daily routine, individuals can better manage the emotional challenges that often accompany trying to conceive.

While alternative approaches to fertility can be beneficial, it is important to remember that they should not replace medical advice or treatment. It is always recommended to consult with a healthcare professional or fertility specialist before incorporating any new practices or supplements into your fertility journey.

Acupuncture for Fertility

Acupuncture is an ancient Chinese practice that involves the insertion of thin needles into specific points on the body. When it comes to fertility, acupuncture has gained popularity as a complementary therapy that may enhance the chances of conceiving.

One of the ways acupuncture may improve fertility is by promoting blood flow to the reproductive organs. By stimulating specific acupuncture points, blood circulation to the uterus and ovaries can be increased, which can enhance the overall health of the reproductive system.

In addition to improving blood flow, acupuncture has also been found to reduce stress levels. The fertility journey can be emotionally challenging, and stress can have a negative impact on fertility. Acupuncture helps to activate the body's relaxation response, reducing stress and creating a more favorable environment for conception.

It's important to note that acupuncture is not a standalone treatment for fertility issues. It is often used in conjunction with other fertility treatments, such as in vitro fertilization (IVF) or intrauterine insemination (IUI). Many fertility clinics offer acupuncture as part of their comprehensive fertility programs.

During an acupuncture session, a licensed acupuncturist will carefully insert thin needles into specific points on your body. The needles are typically left in place for about 20 to 30 minutes, during which you may experience a sense of relaxation and well-being.

It's worth mentioning that acupuncture is generally considered safe when performed by a trained professional. However, it's important to consult with your healthcare provider before starting any new treatments or therapies, especially if you have any underlying medical conditions.

In conclusion, acupuncture may improve fertility by promoting blood flow to the reproductive organs and reducing stress. It can be a valuable addition to your fertility journey, but it's important to remember that individual results may vary. Consult with your healthcare provider to determine if acupuncture is a suitable option for you.

Herbal Supplements for Fertility

Herbal supplements have gained popularity as a natural approach to enhancing fertility. Many people turn to these supplements in the hopes of improving their chances of conceiving. While there is limited scientific evidence to support the effectiveness of these supplements, some individuals have reported positive outcomes. It is important to note that herbal supplements should not replace medical advice or treatment, and consulting with a healthcare professional is essential before incorporating them into your fertility journey.

There are several herbal supplements commonly used to support fertility. Some of the most popular ones include:

- **Vitex:** Also known as chasteberry, vitex is believed to regulate hormone levels and promote regular ovulation. It may be beneficial for women with irregular menstrual cycles.
- **Maca:** Maca root is often used to enhance fertility in both men and women. It is believed to support hormonal balance and improve reproductive health.
- **Raspberry leaf:** Raspberry leaf is commonly used to strengthen the uterus and promote a healthy reproductive system. It is often consumed in the form of tea.
- **Evening primrose oil:** This oil is rich in omega-6 fatty acids, which may support hormonal balance and cervical mucus production.

- **Red clover:** Red clover is believed to have estrogen-like effects, which may help regulate hormone levels and improve fertility.

While these herbal supplements are generally considered safe, it is important to use caution and follow the recommended dosage. Some supplements may interact with medications or have side effects. It is advisable to consult with a healthcare professional before starting any new supplement regimen, especially if you have any underlying health conditions or are taking medications.

It is worth noting that herbal supplements should not be relied upon as a sole solution for fertility issues. They should be used in conjunction with a healthy lifestyle, proper nutrition, and any recommended medical treatments. Remember, every individual's fertility journey is unique, and what works for one person may not work for another. It is always best to seek personalized advice and guidance from a healthcare professional.

Mind-Body Therapies

Mind-body therapies offer a holistic approach to fertility by addressing the connection between the mind and body. These techniques can help reduce stress and promote a positive mindset, which can have a beneficial impact on fertility. Here are some mind-body therapies that you can explore:

- **Yoga:** Practicing yoga can help reduce stress and promote relaxation. Certain yoga poses and sequences are specifically designed to support reproductive health and balance hormones. Additionally, yoga can improve blood flow to the reproductive organs, which can enhance fertility.
- **Meditation:** Meditation is a powerful tool for reducing stress and promoting emotional well-being. By incorporating meditation into your daily routine, you can create a sense of calm and balance, which can positively impact your fertility journey.
- **Visualization:** Visualization involves using your imagination to create mental images of your desired outcome. By visualizing yourself successfully conceiving and carrying a healthy pregnancy, you can cultivate a positive mindset and reduce anxiety. This technique can be combined with meditation for enhanced results.

By incorporating mind-body therapies into your fertility journey, you can create a supportive environment for conception. These techniques can help you manage stress, reduce anxiety, and promote emotional well-being, all of which can positively influence your fertility. Remember to consult with a healthcare professional or fertility specialist to determine which mind-body therapies are suitable for you.

Dealing with Emotional Challenges

Dealing with Emotional Challenges

Trying to conceive can be an emotional roller coaster, filled with ups and downs. It's important to address the emotional aspects of this journey, as they can have a significant impact on your well-being and overall experience. Coping with disappointment, managing anxiety, and seeking support are essential in navigating the emotional challenges that arise.

Coping with Disappointment:

- Understand that it's normal to feel disappointed when conception doesn't happen as quickly as expected.
- Allow yourself to grieve and process your emotions. It's okay to feel sad, frustrated, or even angry.
- Find healthy outlets for your emotions, such as talking to a trusted friend or family member, journaling, or engaging in activities that bring you joy and relaxation.
- Focus on self-care and nurturing yourself during this time. Take time to do things that make you happy and help you relax.
- Stay positive and maintain hope. Remember that everyone's journey is different, and your time will come.

Managing Anxiety:

- Anxiety is a common emotion when trying to conceive, as the process can feel overwhelming and uncertain.
- Practice relaxation techniques such as deep breathing exercises, meditation, or yoga to help reduce anxiety and promote a sense of calm.
- Consider seeking professional help if your anxiety becomes overwhelming or starts to interfere with your daily life. Therapy or counseling can provide valuable support and coping strategies.
- Engage in activities that help you relax and take your mind off the fertility journey, such as hobbies, exercise, or spending time in nature.
- Focus on the present moment and try not to dwell on the future or what-ifs. Take things one step at a time and trust in the process.

Seeking Support:

- Don't hesitate to reach out for support during this challenging time. Talking to loved ones who understand and empathize with your situation can provide immense comfort.
- Consider joining a support group for individuals or couples going through similar fertility struggles. Sharing experiences and emotions with others who can relate can be incredibly helpful.
- Explore the option of fertility counseling, where trained professionals can provide guidance, emotional support, and coping strategies tailored to your specific needs.
- Remember that you are not alone in this journey. There is a vast network of support available to help you navigate the emotional challenges of trying to conceive.

Addressing the emotional aspects of trying to conceive is just as important as addressing the physical aspects. Take care of your emotional well-being, seek support when needed, and remember to be gentle with yourself throughout this journey.

Coping with Disappointment

Trying to conceive can be a rollercoaster of emotions, and it's not uncommon to feel disappointed when your attempts are unsuccessful. Dealing with disappointment is an important part of the fertility journey, and there are strategies you can use to cope with the emotional impact and stay positive.

First and foremost, it's essential to give yourself permission to grieve and acknowledge your feelings. It's normal to feel sad, frustrated, or even angry when you don't achieve the desired outcome. Allow yourself to experience these emotions and don't be too hard on yourself.

One helpful strategy is to find healthy ways to express your emotions. This could involve talking to a trusted friend or family member who can provide a listening ear and offer support. You may also consider joining a support group where you can connect with others who are going through a similar experience. Sharing your feelings with others who understand can be incredibly validating and comforting.

Another important aspect of coping with disappointment is taking care of yourself both physically and emotionally. Engaging in self-care activities can help alleviate stress and boost your overall well-being. This could include activities such as exercise, meditation, journaling, or engaging in hobbies that bring you joy.

It's also crucial to maintain a positive mindset throughout your fertility journey. While it can be challenging, focusing on the things you can control and finding gratitude in other areas of your life can help shift your perspective. Surround yourself with positivity and seek out activities that bring you happiness and fulfillment.

Lastly, don't hesitate to seek professional support if needed. Fertility counseling can be beneficial in helping you navigate the emotional challenges of trying to conceive. A trained therapist can provide guidance, coping strategies, and a safe space to process your emotions.

Remember, coping with disappointment is a personal journey, and it's important to find what works best for you. Be patient with yourself, practice self-compassion, and never lose sight of the hope and resilience that lies within you.

Managing Anxiety

Anxiety and stress can be common emotions experienced during the fertility journey. It is important to find effective techniques to manage these feelings in order to maintain a positive mindset and optimize your chances of conceiving. Here are some strategies that can help:

- **Relaxation exercises:** Engaging in relaxation exercises such as deep breathing, progressive muscle relaxation, and guided imagery can help calm your mind and reduce anxiety. These techniques can be easily incorporated into your daily routine and provide a sense of calmness.
- **Therapy options:** Seeking professional help through therapy can be beneficial in managing anxiety and stress. Cognitive-behavioral therapy (CBT) is a common approach that can help you identify and modify negative thought patterns and develop coping mechanisms to deal with anxiety.

Additionally, there are various other methods you can explore to manage anxiety and stress during your fertility journey. These include:

- **Exercise:** Regular physical activity has been shown to reduce stress and anxiety. Find an exercise routine that you enjoy, whether it's yoga, swimming, or simply going for a walk, and make it a regular part of your routine.
- **Meditation and mindfulness:** Practicing meditation and mindfulness techniques can help you stay present and calm your mind. Apps and online resources are available to guide you through these practices.
- **Support groups:** Connecting with others who are going through a similar journey can provide emotional support and understanding. Joining a support group or seeking online communities can be helpful in managing anxiety.

Remember, it's important to prioritize your mental well-being during the fertility journey. By incorporating relaxation exercises, therapy options, and other stress management techniques into your routine, you can better manage anxiety and stress, allowing yourself to stay positive and focused on your goal of conceiving.

Seeking Support

During the challenging journey of trying to conceive, seeking emotional support is crucial. It is important to remember that you are not alone in this process and that there are resources available to help you navigate the emotional ups and downs.

One of the first sources of support can be your loved ones. Sharing your feelings and experiences with your partner, family, and close friends can provide a sense of comfort and understanding. They can offer a listening ear, offer encouragement, and be a source of strength during this time.

Support groups can also be a valuable resource. Connecting with others who are going through a similar journey can provide a sense of community and understanding. In support groups, you can share your experiences, gain insights from others, and receive emotional support. These groups can be in-person or online, depending on your preference.

Additionally, fertility counseling can be beneficial for individuals and couples struggling with the emotional toll of trying to conceive. Fertility counselors are trained professionals who specialize in providing support and guidance during the fertility journey. They can help you navigate the complex emotions, offer coping strategies, and provide a safe space to express your feelings.

Remember, seeking support is not a sign of weakness, but rather a sign of strength and self-care. It is important to prioritize your emotional well-being as you navigate the challenges of trying to conceive. Reach out to your loved ones, explore support groups, and consider fertility counseling to ensure you have the support you need during this time.

Frequently Asked Questions

- **Q: How can I track my ovulation?**

  A: You can track your ovulation by monitoring changes in your basal body temperature, using ovulation predictor kits, or tracking changes in cervical mucus.

- **Q: Can diet affect fertility?**

  A: Yes, a balanced diet and specific nutrients like folate, iron, and omega-3 fatty acids can support fertility. It's important to eat a variety of fruits, vegetables, whole grains, lean proteins, and healthy fats.

- **Q: Does exercise impact fertility?**

  A: Regular physical activity can enhance fertility. Engaging in moderate exercise, such as brisk walking or swimming, can help regulate hormones and improve overall reproductive health.

- **Q: Can stress affect my chances of getting pregnant?**

  A: Yes, high levels of stress can negatively impact fertility. Managing stress through techniques like meditation, yoga, or deep breathing exercises can help improve your chances of conceiving.

- **Q: Are there substances I should avoid when trying to conceive?**

  A: Yes, it's important to avoid tobacco, alcohol, excessive caffeine, and certain medications that may interfere with fertility. It's best to consult with your healthcare provider for a comprehensive list.

- **Q: What is polycystic ovary syndrome (PCOS)?**

  A: PCOS is a common condition that can cause infertility. It is characterized by hormonal imbalances, cysts on the ovaries, and irregular menstrual cycles. Treatment options are available to manage PCOS and improve fertility.

- **Q: How does endometriosis affect fertility?**

  A: Endometriosis can affect fertility by causing inflammation, scarring, and the formation of adhesions in the reproductive organs. Treatment options, such as medication or surgery, can help manage the condition and improve fertility.

- **Q: When should I seek medical help for fertility issues?**

  A: If you have been actively trying to conceive for a year without success (or six months if you're over 35), it's recommended to consult a fertility specialist. They can evaluate your reproductive health and provide appropriate guidance.

- **Q: What are common causes of female infertility?**

A: Female infertility can be caused by ovulation disorders, fallopian tube blockages, uterine abnormalities, or hormonal imbalances. A thorough evaluation by a fertility specialist can help determine the underlying cause.

- **Q: What factors contribute to male infertility?**

A: Male infertility can be caused by sperm abnormalities, hormonal imbalances, genetic conditions, or lifestyle factors such as smoking or excessive alcohol consumption. A fertility specialist can conduct tests to identify potential issues.

- **Q: What are the different fertility treatment options available?**

A: Fertility treatments include medications to stimulate ovulation, intrauterine insemination (IUI) to place sperm directly into the uterus, and in vitro fertilization (IVF) where fertilization occurs outside the body. The most suitable option depends on individual circumstances.

- **Q: Can alternative approaches like acupuncture or herbal supplements enhance fertility?**

A: Some individuals find that alternative approaches like acupuncture, herbal supplements, or mind-body therapies can support their fertility journey. However, it's important to discuss these options with a healthcare provider and ensure their safety and effectiveness.

- **Q: How can I cope with the emotional challenges of trying to conceive?**

A: Coping with disappointment and managing anxiety are important aspects of the fertility journey. Strategies such as seeking emotional support from loved ones, practicing relaxation techniques, or considering therapy can be helpful.

Have Questions / Comments?

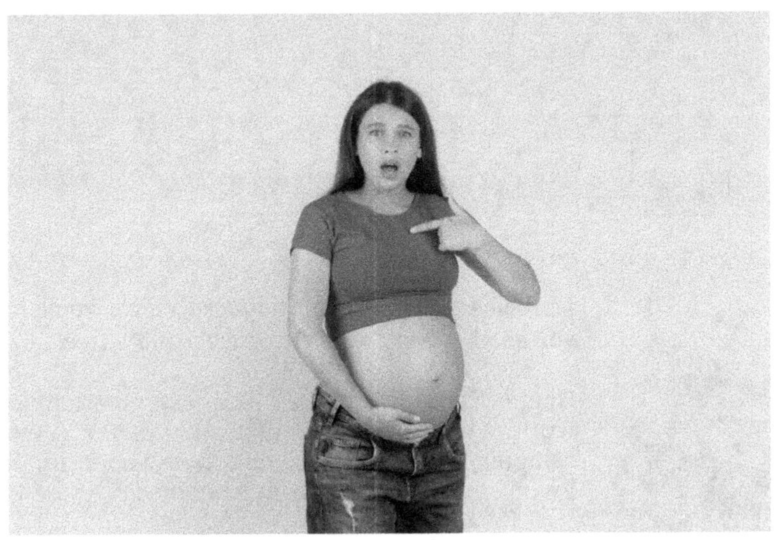

This book was designed to cover as much info as possible but I know I have probably missed something, or some new amazing discovery that has just come out.

If you notice something missing or have a question that I failed to answer, please get in touch and let me know. If I can, I will email you an answer and also update the book so others can also benefit from it.

Thanks For Being Awesome :)

Submit Your Questions / Comments At:
Get In Touch Babydreamers.net

Get How To Be A Super Mom 100% FREE

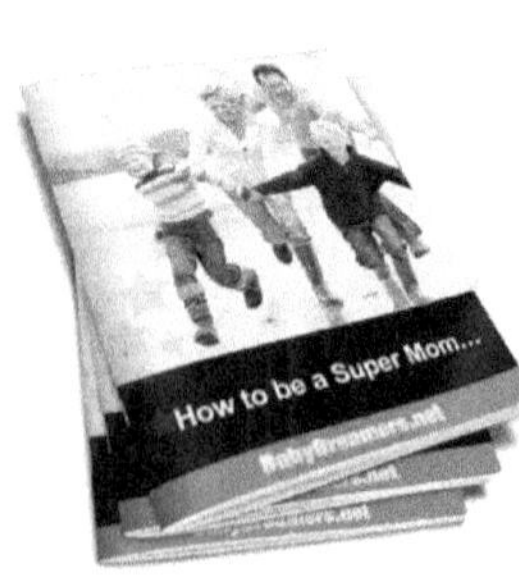

For being one of our amazing readers, we would love to offer you another book we have created, 100% free.

Being a mom is probably the most important job in the world – we've all heard that, and it's true. You're bringing up the next generation of wonderful, intelligent, loving, creative, responsible people.

We all want to be Super Mom and to be everything and do everything, but it this possible?

Being a Super Mom is possible, but you have to learn how to empower yourself to be the kind of Super Mom that you feel you need to be, keeping in mind that the title Super Mom doesn't mean the same thing to everyone.

Get How to be a Super Mom For Free